CHAIR YOGA FOR MEN OVER 50

The Ultimate Guide For Older People To Lose Weight, Build Strength, Enhance Mobility, Flexibility And Balance With Simple Daily Chair Exercises

Silvanus Bekee

Table of Contents

INTRODUCTION

In a world constantly buzzing with activity, finding solace and rejuvenation becomes paramount, especially as we gracefully age. Imagine this: A seasoned gentleman, perhaps in his 50s, embarks on a journey to rediscover vitality and well-being. Faced with the inevitable changes that accompany aging, he stumbles upon a transformative practice 'Chair Yoga'. Little did he know that this guide would become his compass, leading him to a realm where mind, body, and spirit unite in harmonious balance.

As the pages of this guide unfold, our protagonist discovers a profound sense of liberation within the confines of a chair. In a society often fixated on high-intensity workouts, Chair Yoga emerges as a beacon of inclusivity, embracing men over 50 with open arms. Through gentle movements, breath work, and mindful poses, the guide becomes a roadmap to resilience, cultivating strength, flexibility, and peace of mind. This journey is not just about physical wellness; it's a holistic expedition into the realms of mental clarity and emotional serenity.

The benefits of Chair Yoga for men over 50 extend far beyond the physical. Picture our protagonist reclaiming his mornings with increased energy, gracefully navigating the challenges of daily life with newfound agility, and cultivating a sense of calm that permeates every aspect of his being. The guide becomes a trusted companion, seamlessly integrating into his routine, fostering a resilient foundation that defies the limitations often associated with aging.

Join us on this transformative odyssey as we delve into the intricacies of Chair Yoga, unveiling a holistic approach to wellness tailored specifically for men over 50. It's time to embrace the power of the chair, rediscover the joy of movement, and embark on a journey towards a healthier, more vibrant life.

CHAPTER 1

Understanding Chair Yoga

Chair Yoga is a gentle and accessible form of yoga that caters to a diverse audience, offering a seated practice designed to accommodate individuals with varying physical abilities. Rooted in traditional yoga principles, this modified approach utilizes a chair as a supportive prop, making it an ideal option for those who may face challenges with mobility or prefer a seated practice.

Understanding Chair Yoga involves recognizing its versatility in adapting classic yoga postures to a seated or partially seated position, promoting accessibility for individuals of all ages and fitness levels. The practice focuses on cultivating mindfulness, breath awareness, and gentle movements that enhance flexibility, strength, and balance. It becomes an inclusive avenue for seniors, those recovering from injuries, or anyone seeking a less strenuous yet beneficial form of exercise.

Chair Yoga emphasizes the mind-body connection, encouraging practitioners to center themselves through conscious breathing and intentional movements. Beyond physical benefits, it fosters emotional well-being and a sense of calm. Whether in an office setting, community center, or home environment, grasping the essence of Chair Yoga involves appreciating its adaptability and the potential to bring the transformative power of yoga to a broader spectrum of individuals, fostering a holistic approach to wellness.

Core Benefits Of Chair Yoga For Men Over 50

1. Enhanced Flexibility: The guide introduces tailored Chair Yoga poses that gently stretch and improve flexibility, ensuring a gradual increase in range of motion for men over 50.

2. Improved Strength: Through strategic chair-based exercises, the guide targets key muscle groups, fostering increased strength and stability for daily activities.

3. Joint Health: Gentle movements promote joint mobility, reducing stiffness and enhancing overall joint health, particularly beneficial for those experiencing age-related challenges.

4. Stress Reduction: Incorporating mindful breathing techniques and relaxation poses, the guide provides a sanctuary for men over 50 to alleviate stress and cultivate a tranquil state of mind.

5. Better Posture: Addressing common posture concerns associated with aging, the guide focuses on exercises that promote spine alignment and core strength, aiding in improved posture.

6. Increased Energy Levels: By stimulating circulation and incorporating energizing sequences, the guide becomes a catalyst for boosting energy levels, empowering users to tackle daily tasks with vigor.

7. Enhanced Balance: The program incorporates balance-focused poses to help counterbalance the effects of aging, reducing the risk of falls and promoting stability.

8. Mind-Body Connection: Chair Yoga encourages a mindful connection between body and breath, fostering a sense of presence and mindfulness that extends beyond the yoga practice.

9. Adaptability: Tailored to the needs of men over 50, the guide offers modifications and variations, ensuring accessibility for individuals with varying fitness levels and physical conditions.

10. Holistic Wellness: Beyond physical benefits, the guide addresses mental and emotional well-being, providing a holistic approach to health that encompasses the mind, body, and spirit, promoting a balanced and fulfilling life.

Safety Precautions And Guidelines

1. Consultation with Healthcare Professional: Before starting any exercise program, especially if you have pre-existing health conditions, it is advisable to consult with a healthcare professional to ensure Chair Yoga is suitable for your individual needs.

2. Chair Stability: Use a sturdy, non-slip chair with a backrest and ensure it is placed on a flat surface. Avoid using chairs with wheels or instability to prevent accidents during the practice.

3. Awareness of Physical Limits: Listen to your body and avoid pushing yourself too hard. Modify poses as needed, and refrain from movements that cause discomfort or pain. Gradually progress to more challenging poses over time.

4. Warm-Up and Cool Down: Always begin with a gentle warm-up to prepare your body for movement and end with a cool-down to promote flexibility and prevent muscle strain.

5. Proper Breathing Techniques: Focus on controlled, mindful breathing throughout the practice. Avoid breath-holding and ensure a steady flow of breath to enhance relaxation and oxygenation.

6. Comfortable Clothing: Wear comfortable, breathable clothing that allows for a full range of motion. Avoid overly loose or restrictive attire that may impede movement or compromise safety.

7. Secure Environment: Practice in a well-lit, clutter-free space to minimize the risk of tripping or bumping into objects. Ensure the area around your chair is free of hazards.

8. Hydration: Stay adequately hydrated before, during, and after your practice. Dehydration can exacerbate muscle stiffness and increase the risk of injury.

9. Personalized Modifications: Adapt poses and exercises to your individual needs and abilities. If you have specific health concerns, work with a qualified instructor to tailor the practice to your requirements.

10. Regular Check-ins: Periodically reassess your fitness level and any changes in your health. Modify your practice accordingly and stay attuned to your body's signals for a safe and enjoyable Chair Yoga experience.

WARM UP EXERCISES

1. Seated Neck Rolls:

- Sit comfortably in the chair with your back straight.

- Slowly lower your chin towards your chest, then gently roll your head to one side, bringing your ear towards your shoulder.

- Continue the circular motion, moving your head to the opposite side and back to the starting position.

- Repeat the sequence, alternating directions. This exercise helps release tension in the neck and shoulders.

2. Shoulder Shrugs:

- In a seated position, inhale as you raise both shoulders towards your ears.

- Exhale as you relax and lower your shoulders.

- Repeat this movement for 10-15 reps, promoting flexibility and releasing tension in the shoulder muscles.

3. Seated Cat-Cow Stretch:

- Sit with your feet flat on the floor, hands resting on your knees.

- Inhale, arch your back, and lift your chest (Cow Stretch).

- Exhale, round your spine, and bring your chin towards your chest (Cat Stretch).

- Repeat this flowing movement, synchronizing breath with motion to warm up the spine.

4. Ankle Circles:

- Extend one leg and rotate your ankle in a circular motion.

- Perform 10 circles in one direction, then switch to the other leg.

- This exercise promotes ankle flexibility and helps improve circulation in the lower extremities.

5. Seated Side Bends:

- Sit with your feet flat on the floor and your hands resting on your thighs.
- Inhale as you lengthen your spine, then exhale as you gently lean to one side, reaching towards the floor.

- Inhale back to the center, then exhale to the opposite side.

- Repeat for 8-10 reps on each side to stretch the sides of the torso.

CHAPTER 2

CHAIR YOGA

1. Seated Knee Lifts:

- Starting Position:
Sit tall in the chair with feet flat on the floor.

- Steps:
1. Inhale, lifting one knee towards your chest.
2. Exhale, gently lowering the foot back to the floor.
3. Repeat on the other leg.

- Repetitions:
Perform 10-12 lifts on each leg.

- Purpose:
Strengthens the hip flexors and improves leg mobility.

2. Chair Mountain Pose:

- Starting Position:

Sit comfortably with feet hip-width apart and hands resting on thighs.

- Steps:

1. Inhale, reaching arms overhead, palms facing each other.

2. Exhale, bringing hands back to thighs.

- Repetitions:

Repeat 8-10 times.

- Purpose:

Enhances overall posture, stretches the spine, and engages core muscles.

3. Seated Forward Fold:

- Starting Position:

Sit with legs extended straight in front.

- Steps:

1. Inhale, lengthening the spine.
2. Exhale, hinge at the hips, reaching towards your toes.

- Repetitions:

Hold for 15-20 seconds, repeating 3 times.

- Purpose:

Stretches the hamstrings, lower back, and promotes flexibility.

4. Seated Twist:

- Starting Position:

Sit tall, cross one leg over the other.

- Steps:

1. Inhale, lengthening the spine.

2. Exhale, twisting towards the crossed leg.

- Repetitions:

Hold for 15-20 seconds, alternating sides.

- Purpose:

Improves spinal mobility and releases tension in the back.

5. Chair Warrior Pose:

- Starting Position:

Sit at the front edge of the chair, one leg extended back.

- Steps:

1. Inhale, reaching arms overhead.

2. Exhale, engaging the core and leaning slightly forward.

- Repetitions:

Hold for 20-30 seconds, switch legs, and repeat.

- Purpose:

Strengthens the legs, improves balance, and stretches the arms and back.

6. Seated Leg Extensions:

- Starting Position:

Sit upright with feet flat on the floor.

- Steps:

1. Inhale, extend one leg straight in front.
2. Exhale, lower the leg back down.

- Repetitions:

Perform 12-15 extensions on each leg.

- Purpose:

Targets quadriceps and improves lower body strength.

7. Seated Chest Opener:

- Starting Position:

Sit with a straight back, hands clasped behind your back.

- Steps:

1. Inhale, lift the chest and gently squeeze the shoulder blades together.

2. Exhale, releasing the arms and relaxing the shoulders.

- Repetitions:

Repeat 8-10 times.

- Purpose:

Opens the chest, stretches the shoulders, and promotes better posture.

8. Seated Leg Cross Stretch:

- Starting Position:

Sit with legs crossed, one ankle over the opposite knee.

- Steps:

1. Inhale, lengthening the spine.

2. Exhale, gently leaning forward to feel a stretch in the outer hip.

- Repetitions:

Hold for 15-20 seconds, switch legs, and repeat.

- Purpose:

Stretches the hips and glutes, improving flexibility.

9. Chair Side Leg Lifts:

- Starting Position:

Sit with feet flat on the floor and hands resting on the sides of the chair.

- Steps:

1. Inhale, lift one leg to the side.
2. Exhale, lower the leg back down.

- Repetitions:

Perform 10-12 lifts on each leg.

- Purpose:

Targets the outer thighs, improving leg strength and stability.

10. Seated Bicep Curls:

- Starting Position:

Sit with a straight back, holding light dumbbells in each hand.

- Steps:

1. Inhale, curl the weights towards your shoulders.
2. Exhale, lower the weights back down.

- Repetitions:

Repeat for 12-15 curls.

- Purpose:

Strengthens the biceps and forearms, enhancing upper body strength.

11. Seated Hip Flexor Stretch:

- Starting Position:

Sit tall with one-foot flat on the floor and the opposite ankle crossed over the knee.

- Steps:

1. Inhale, lengthen the spine.

2. Exhale, gently lean forward, feeling a stretch in the hip of the crossed leg.

- Repetitions:

Hold for 15-20 seconds, switch legs, and repeat.

- Purpose:

Releases tension in the hip flexors, promoting flexibility.

12. Seated Wrist and Forearm Stretch:

- Starting Position:

Sit with a straight back, extend one arm forward with palm facing down.

- Steps:

1. Inhale, gently press down on the fingers with the opposite hand.

2. Exhale, feeling a stretch in the wrist and forearm.

- Repetitions:

Hold for 15-20 seconds on each arm.

- Purpose:

Alleviates tension in the wrists and forearms, beneficial for those with desk-related strain.

13. Seated Knee to Chest Stretch:

- Starting Position:

Sit with feet flat on the floor.

- Steps:

1. Inhale, lift one knee towards the chest, hugging it with both hands.

2. Exhale, gently release the leg back down.

- Repetitions:

Perform 10-12 stretches on each leg.

- Purpose:

Stretches the lower back and hips, improving flexibility.

14. Seated Ankle Flex and Point:

- Starting Position:

Sit with feet flat on the floor.

- Steps:

1. Inhale, flex both ankles, bringing toes towards you.
2. Exhale, point both ankles away from you.

- Repetitions:

Repeat for 15-20 flex-and-point cycles.

- Purpose:

Enhances ankle mobility and improves circulation in the lower legs.

15. Chair Child's Pose Variation:

- Starting Position:

Sit with knees wide and toes touching, leaning forward with arms extended on the chair.

- Steps:

1. Inhale, lengthen the spine.

2. Exhale, sink back into the stretch, reaching arms further forward.

- Repetitions:

Hold for 20-30 seconds, repeating 2-3 times.

- Purpose:

Relaxes the back, shoulders, and promotes a sense of calm and release.

16. Seated Calf Raises:

- Starting Position:

Sit with feet flat on the floor.

- Steps:

1. Inhale, lift both heels off the ground.
2. Exhale, lower the heels back down.

- Repetitions:

Perform 15-20 calf raises.

- Purpose:

Strengthens the calf muscles and promotes ankle stability.

17. Seated Side Stretch:

- Starting Position:

Sit tall with feet flat on the floor.

- Steps:

1. Inhale, raise one arm overhead.

2. Exhale, gently lean to the opposite side.

- Repetitions:

Hold for 15-20 seconds on each side.

- Purpose:

Stretches the sides of the torso, promoting lateral flexibility.

18. Seated Clasped Hands Twist:

- Starting Position:

Sit tall with feet flat on the floor, clasp hands in front of you.

- Steps:

1. Inhale, lengthen the spine.

2. Exhale, twist to one side, using the clasped hands for support.

- Repetitions:

Hold for 15-20 seconds, switch sides, and repeat.

- Purpose:

Improves spinal mobility and stretches the back and shoulders.

19. Seated Hamstring Stretch with Strap:

- Starting Position:

Sit with legs extended and a strap around one foot.

- Steps:

1. Inhale, lengthen the spine.

2. Exhale, gently hinge at the hips, using the strap to pull the foot towards you.

- Repetitions:

Hold for 20-30 seconds, switch legs, and repeat.

- Purpose:

Deepens the hamstring stretch with added support.

20. Seated Diaphragmatic Breathing:

- **Starting Position:**

Sit comfortably, placing one hand on the chest and the other on the abdomen.

- **Steps:**

1. Inhale deeply through the nose, expanding the diaphragm.

2. Exhale slowly through pursed lips, engaging the abdominal muscles.

- **Repetitions:**

Practice for 5-10 minutes.

- **Purpose:**

Promotes relaxation, reduces stress, and enhances respiratory function.

21. Seated Quadriceps Stretch:

- Starting Position:

Sit on the edge of the chair with feet hip-width apart.

- Steps:

1. Inhale, lift one foot towards the buttocks, holding the ankle.

2. Exhale, gently press the foot towards the buttocks.

- Repetitions:

Hold for 15-20 seconds on each leg.

- Purpose:

Stretches the front of the thigh, improving quadriceps flexibility.

22. Seated Figure Four Stretch:

- Starting Position:

Sit tall with feet flat on the floor.

- Steps:

1. Cross one ankle over the opposite knee.

2. Inhale, lengthen the spine, and exhale, gently leaning forward.

- Repetitions:

Hold for 15-20 seconds, switch legs, and repeat.

- Purpose:

Stretches the hips and glutes, promoting flexibility.

23. Seated Wrist Circles:

- Starting Position:

Sit with a straight back, extend arms in front.

- Steps:

1. Rotate wrists in a circular motion, first in one direction, then the other.

- Repetitions:

Perform 10-15 circles in each direction.

- Purpose:

Enhances wrist mobility and alleviates tension.

24. Chair Warrior II Pose:

- Starting Position:

Sit at the front edge of the chair with feet wide.

- Steps:

1. Inhale, extend arms parallel to the floor, facing forward.

2. Exhale, gently twist the torso to one side.

- Repetitions:

Hold for 20-30 seconds, switch sides, and repeat.

- Purpose:

Strengthens the legs, improves balance, and stretches the torso.

25. Seated Side Leg Circles:

- Starting Position:

Sit with feet flat on the floor.

- Steps:

1. Lift one leg slightly and draw small circles with the toes.

2. Reverse the direction of the circles.

- Repetitions:

Perform 10-15 circles in each direction on each leg.

- Purpose:

Enhances hip mobility and engages the leg muscles.

26. Seated Triceps Dips:

- Starting Position:

Sit on the edge of the chair with hands gripping the sides.

- Steps:

1. Inhale, lift your body off the chair by straightening your arms.

2. Exhale, lower your body back down without fully sitting.

- Repetitions:

Perform 12-15 triceps dips.

- Purpose:

Strengthens the triceps and improves arm tone.

27. Seated Bicycle Crunches:

- Starting Position:

Sit with feet flat on the floor, hands behind your head.

- Steps:

1. Inhale, lift one knee towards your chest while twisting your torso to touch the opposite elbow.

2. Exhale, switch to the other knee and elbow.

- Repetitions:

Perform 15-20 bicycle crunches on each side.

- Purpose:

Engages the core muscles and promotes abdominal strength.

28. Seated Eagle Arms:

- Starting Position:

Sit tall with arms extended in front.

- Steps:

1. Cross one arm over the other, bringing palms together.
2. Inhale, lift the elbows while lowering the shoulders.

- Repetitions:

Hold for 15-20 seconds, switch arm positions, and repeat.

- Purpose:

Stretches the upper back and shoulders, improving flexibility.

29. Seated Pelvic Tilts:

- Starting Position:

Sit with a straight back and feet flat on the floor.

- Steps:

1. Inhale, arch your lower back and tilt your pelvis forward.

2. Exhale, round your lower back and tilt your pelvis backward.

- Repetitions:

Perform 12-15 pelvic tilts.

- Purpose:

Promotes flexibility in the spine and strengthens the core.

30. Seated Ankle Alphabet:

- Starting Position:

Sit with feet flat on the floor.

- Steps:

1. Lift one foot slightly and trace the alphabet with your toes.

2. Switch to the other foot.

- Repetitions:

Complete the alphabet with each foot.

- Purpose:

Improves ankle mobility and enhances coordination.

SPECIAL MOTIVATIONAL QUOTES

1. "Embrace the strength within your seated sanctuary. Chair yoga for men over 50 is not just a practice; it's a journey of resilience, proving that every mindful breath and gentle stretch carries the power to transform and renew."

2. "In the realm of the chair, discover the warrior within. Age is not a limitation but a canvas for new beginnings. With each seated pose, weave a tapestry of strength, flexibility, and the unwavering spirit of possibility."

3. "Chair yoga for men over 50 is a testament to the wisdom that resides in stillness. As you flow within the confines of your seat, remember: The power to rejuvenate is not bound by time; it is found in the commitment to your own well-being."

4. "Seated strength knows no boundaries. In the embrace of the chair, let every movement be a declaration: 'I am here, resilient and evolving.' The journey of chair yoga for men over 50 is not about limits; it's about rewriting possibilities."

5. "Your chair is not a throne of limitation but a seat of empowerment. In the world of chair yoga, let each breath be a reminder that age is not a countdown but a celebration of the unwritten chapters of strength and vitality."

CONCLUSION

In conclusion, Chair Yoga emerges as a holistic and transformative practice tailored specifically for men over 50, proving that the journey to well-being knows no age-related boundaries. Through a symphony of mindful breath work, gentle movements, and adapted poses, this seated discipline becomes a gateway to enhanced flexibility, strength, and emotional equilibrium. The chair, once seen as a symbol of rest, transforms into a vessel of empowerment, supporting a renewed sense of vitality and resilience.

As we navigate the realms of seated poses and soothing stretches, the essence of Chair Yoga transcends the physical; it becomes a sanctuary for the mind, an oasis of calm amidst life's demands. It's a journey of self-discovery, an exploration of one's own body and its incredible capacity for rejuvenation. The wisdom gained from this practice is not merely about the postures but about embracing the present moment and finding harmony within the constraints of a seated position.

For every man over 50 embarking on this venture, remember: Your journey is unique, and your potential is boundless. In the gentle ebb and flow of chair yoga, recognize the strength that resides within you. It's a strength that defies expectations, transcends limitations, and redefines what it means to age gracefully. As you commit to this path of well-being, let each seated breath be a whisper of encouragement, a reminder that you possess the power to nurture your body, mind, and spirit.

So, with the chair as your ally, continue this journey with confidence and purpose. Let the wisdom of chair yoga infuse your life with renewed energy and a profound sense of well-being.

FITNESS

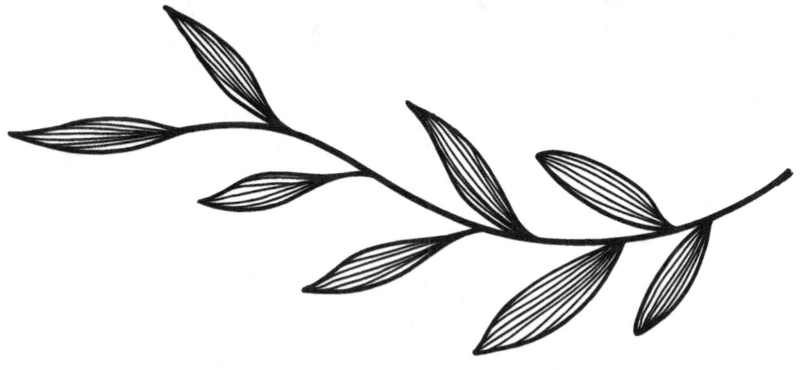

PLANNER

Fitness Planner

NAME: **DATE:**

BREAKFAST

LUNCH

DINNER

SNACK

EXERCISE	SET	REP	NOTES

Fitness Planner

NAME: **DATE:**

BREAKFAST

LUNCH

DINNER

SNACK

EXERCISE	SET	REP	NOTES

Fitness Planner

NAME:

DATE:

BREAKFAST

LUNCH

DINNER

SNACK

EXERCISE

SET

REP

NOTES

Fitness Planner

NAME: **DATE:**

BREAKFAST

LUNCH

DINNER

SNACK

EXERCISE   SET   REP   NOTES

Fitness Planner

NAME:

DATE:

BREAKFAST

LUNCH

DINNER

SNACK

EXERCISE

SET

REP

NOTES

Fitness Planner

NAME: **DATE:**

BREAKFAST   LUNCH

DINNER   SNACK

EXERCISE   SET   REP   NOTES

Fitness Planner

NAME: **DATE:**

BREAKFAST

LUNCH

DINNER

SNACK

EXERCISE | SET | REP | NOTES

Fitness Planner

NAME: **DATE:**

BREAKFAST

LUNCH

DINNER

SNACK

EXERCISE   SET   REP   NOTES

Fitness Planner

NAME: DATE:

BREAKFAST

LUNCH

DINNER

SNACK

EXERCISE	SET	REP	NOTES

Fitness Planner

NAME: **DATE:**

BREAKFAST

LUNCH

DINNER

SNACK

EXERCISE   SET   REP   NOTES